The Ketogenic

A Deliciously Satisfying Eating Plan To Lose Weight, Flatten Your Belly and Feel Great

By: Jennifer Williams

ISBN-13:978-1490932385

TABLE OF CONTENTS

PUBLISHERS NOTES

Disclaimer

Paperback Edition

Manufactured in the United States of America

INTRODUCTION

So, if you are like many of us that are about to engage on a new weight loss diet, you are wondering what you many have gotten yourself in to and if *this one* will be the diet that will give you results.

First and foremost, the initiative you are taking to start a new plan to lose weight is an important step. You have recognized that you need to do something (whatever that something is) to improve your eating habits and health. So pat yourself on the back and get ready to dive in.

My goal with this book is to answer your questions about what the Ketogenic Diet is, how you can go about fitting this diet into your lifestyle and eating habits, and what outcomes you can expect to achieve.

Simply stated the Ketogenic Diet entails eating fewer (or no) carbohydrates while increasing your healthy fats and proteins. You've most certainly have heard of low carb diets such as Atkins, South Beach, Paleo and the intermittent-type diets such as the 5:2 Diet.

The basic tenets of these diets are that eating healthier and, more specifically, eating foods that have low carbohydrates and higher proteins are just great for fat loss.

One such form of this type of dieting that has been practiced for many centuries now is simply known as – Fasting. The important thing to note about this age old diet is that it was practiced mainly for reasons such as abstinence and a theoretical belief in purity.

After much research on the subject of Fasting, many biological processes that were at work during Fasting came to be understood. What was discovered was that the very same biological results were obtained with Fasting, as were obtained with a carbohydrate free diet.

Plus, it was also found that by restricting the carbs in the diet, it was actually possible to achieve quick weight loss.

There are fans and opponents to all of these diets. Actually for most diets, there are those that swear by the results and those that question the science and the benefits of these diets. This is no different for the Ketogenic Diet.

There are actually 3 forms of the Ketogenic Diet; the Standard form which restricts all carbohydrates; the Targeted Ketogenic Diet which allows for eating carbohydrates around exercise; and the Cyclical Ketogenic Diet which alternates extended days of high carbohydrate consumption with days of Ketogenic Dieting that maintain ketosis.

What this book will do is explain to you, in the easiest way possible, the physiology that supports this type of diet, the results you can achieve in weight loss and how you feel, and how you can implement this diet to achieve the best results for you.

CHAPTER 1- THE SCIENCE BEHIND THE DIET

So Just How Does The Ketogenic Diet Work?

As you know, in order for your body to be able to function, it requires a regular supply of fuel. For this fuel, your body, your brain, your muscles and all the organs in your body will either make use of glucose or ketones as a source of fuel supply.

With most eating habits, your body consumes a mix of carbohydrates, proteins and fats for fuel. However, when you remove carbohydrates from your diet, your body is forced to find alternative sources to fuel your systems.

The foundation of the Ketogenic diet is that we can cause our body to burn greater amounts of fat by decreasing its use of glucose, which comes from carbohydrates.

Now, what you need to understand here is that it is the function of the pancreas and the liver to regulate the fuel supply to the body. And the fact is that the liver and the pancreas prefer to generate this fuel supply from glucose.

The reason why glucose is the preferred source for supply of fuel to the body is due to the fact that it is very easily available from stores in the muscles and also it is readily available in the liver. Plus, glucose is found in abundance from many of the foods that you eat.

On the other hand it is not easy for ketones to be used as a fuel source as they have to be forcefully synthesized by the liver. Whereas, the liver synthesizes glucose very easily and without any force.

In very simple words – when you embark on this diet, you will encourage your body to make use of your very own body fat stores as the primary source of energy - instead of your body making use of carbohydrates as the primary source for energy. The latter is what is normally done when you eat carbohydrates and simple sugars.

The bottom-line is that that you will be able to lose excess fat and inches very quickly by eating nutritious foods with the appropriate balance of fats, proteins and carbohydrates.

When Your Body Gets Carbs And When It Does Not Get Carbs

You need to know how this diet works to get it to work well for you. Therefore, the first thing you must understand is what happens when your body gets carbohydrates and when it does not get carbohydrates.

When your body gets an intake of carbs, there is a resultant spike of insulin that takes place in your body. This actually means that your pancreas is releasing insulin. Thus, common sense will tell you that if you stop having carbs, then the insulin will not store excess calories in the form of fats. And this is an ideal situation.

So, now that your body does not have carbs to give you a supply of energy, it needs to find a new source of energy. And this new source of energy is – Fat!

Just What Your Body Needs To Lose Weight

Yes, this is just what is required for you to lose your body fat! When your body does not get carbs, it will start breaking down the fats that are present in your body and make use of these fats as a source of energy.

And this state is defined to be as - Ketosis. Ketosis is the shift your body makes from metabolizing glucose to metabolizing fat to fuel your body. This is just the state that you want your body to be in so that you can lose your excess body fat, while at the same time maintain muscle.

Why The Big Fuss For Ketones When Glucose Is Readily Available?

You would be very right in asking this question. Why go through all the trouble of forcing your body to use ketones as a source of fuel, when glucose is available so readily? The reason why it is good for the body to use ketones is that when the body starts to use ketones instead of glucose as a fuel source, the following great stuff starts to happen to your body:

1. The energy level of the body gets to a state that is not only very high, but it also becomes very stable.
2. Muscle loss is reduced greatly.
3. Breakdown of body fats increases vastly.
4. Elimination of water retention takes place.

This is what happens when your body arrives at a state of Ketosis. As you can see there are many benefits to the body being in the state of Ketosis. In this state, your body will be making use of fat in the form of ketones, to supply all the fuel that your body needs.

This is really good for your body as in this way, your body is not going to break up the muscles. This is because now in this way the muscles have nothing to offer and the body only needs fats (at least to a larger extent). And for any dieter this is great news as this means much less muscle loss and higher energy, compared to many other weight loss diets.

CHAPTER 2- WHAT MAKES THIS DIET WORK

Many dieters and diet books focus purely on total weight loss. This is understandable since we have been conditioned to measure our dieting progress by looking at the numbers on our scales. How many magazines covers have you seen that tout the 'lose 10 pounds in a week' diets? However, this does not paint the true picture of our healthy body weight.

Many diets, the Ketogenic Diet included, can result in rapid weight loss in the initial days. Why? Water! Water weight is the initial pounds that are released in many of these high intensity diets.

While water weight loss is a good first step and makes many dieters feel great about their early progress, it is also the reason many dieters fail. First after the initial water loss, the next tier of weight loss is slightly slower – many dieters by this point find it difficult to stay on their diet. Secondly, while water is the easiest thing to lose, it is also the easiest to add back on to your weight – thus many dieters see this as a failure of their diet

What a dieter needs to focus on to 'truly' lose weight is not the overall weight, but the composition of body fat to total body weight. Fat, muscle and water make up our total body weight. What you as a dieter really want is fat loss. When you restrict calories but do not know where the weight loss is coming from, you do not know if you are accomplishing your ultimate goals – to lose fat.

Another critical factor in dieting is our metabolic rate. This is the amount of energy our body utilizes to maintain normal functions plus any additional activities. When we consume more that we use, we gain weight. So if we want to lose weight, we either reduce our calories consumed or increase our activity levels or ideally some balance of both.

Ideally we need to find the optimum amount of calories to consume based upon our energy use. This not unlike what most diets tell you: reduce your calories and exercise more. Unfortunately, what we have a tendency to do is to restrict our calories to the extreme.

When we severely restrict our calories, our metabolic rate decreases (sometimes as much 30 percent or more). Consequently, our energy expenditure also decreases causing less weight loss than anticipated. Extreme calorie reduction can also result in muscle loss instead of our desired fat loss.

What This Means To You

When people talk about a Ketogenic Diet they are typically referring to the Standard Ketogenic Diet (SKD). This form of the diet is low in carbohydrates and moderately high in fats and proteins.

There are two typically seen modifications of the Standard Ketogenic Diet; the Targeted Ketogenic Diet (TKD) which allows for higher carb consumption around intense periods of exercise, and the Cyclical Ketogenic Diet (CKD) which cycles 5 days on and 2 days off of low carb consumption. The CKD is frequently used by bodybuilders.

There are also of course many modifications that others have made and you too can make to this diet. Do what suits both your activity levels, how much fat you want to lose and what works well for your body type and lifestyle.

The Ketogenic Diet

Our intent is to give you plenty of information about the basics behind the Ketogenic Diet and then suggest foods and meal plans to help you find what works best for you.

If you understand the basics, get a good start and some great early results, there is a much greater likelihood that you will continue your diet. Once you start to look and feel better, you will feel very satisfied with what you are eating and be able to stick to the diet.

CHAPTER 3- THE TYPES OF FOODS YOU CAN EAT

The Ketogenic Diet is highly effective if you want to get quick, ultra-low, body fat levels, while at the same time having maximum muscle retention.

If this diet is done in the way that it is meant to be done, the kind of fat loss and reduced inches that you will experience is extremely satisfying and motivating. Plus, you will find that you will have extremely high energy levels and a tremendous sense of well-being, overall.

The primary components of the Ketogenic Diet are consume *more Proteins and Fats* and *fewer or no Carbohydrates*.

Protein Is A Must

With this diet, every meal contains protein. Protein is a must as this helps in reducing your appetite and also, it helps in preserving lean muscle mass, as well as in the regulation of the blood glucose levels. Excellent examples of foods that contain proteins are: **meat, eggs, turkey, chicken, cheese, pork and fish**, to name a few foods.

It is also a great idea to consume drinks that are rich in protein such as soy protein or whey protein isolate. Soy protein is very good as it can reduce fat levels and it also promotes fat loss. Soy protein has the ability to do this as it contains essential fatty acids and phyto-estrogens that promote fat loss.

But, at the same time while on this diet, it is important that your body gets balanced nutrition, including fiber, minerals, and vitamins and it is also vital that your body promotes detoxification. So, it is imperative that you have at least 3 or 4 **cups of veggies that have**

low carbohydrate content or a salad – and that too on a daily basis. You could also have an optional serving of **fresh fruit**.

Carbohydrates – What To Eliminate

This Ketogenic Diet calls for eliminating or significantly reducing carbohydrates. However, there are good carbs and bad carbs. We only really need to get rid of the bad, or simple, carbs. While not trying to make this diet any more difficult to understand, we think this is an important distinction. As you will see in the example meal plans and foods that we talk about later, there are carbohydrates in several of these foods – but those are the good carbs.

Good carbs are also known as *complex carbohydrates*. Complex carbohydrates are the *right kind of carbs* to eat. Complex carbohydrates, because of their higher fiber and chemical structure, make our bodies work harder to digest them and then their energy is released over a longer period of time.

The Ketogenic Diet requires the elimination of *simple carbs* or *bad carbs*. Simple carbohydrates are sugars that are easily digested and stored in our bodies as glycogen. If these are not immediately used by our body, they are converted to fat.

Bad carbs are usually found in processed foods, foods that have been stripped of their natural fibers and nutrients, and sugars.

Watch Out For Sugar

One of the worst contributors to excess fat and increased health problems is sugar. You have most likely read hundreds of times to avoid or reduce your sugar consumption. But do you know the many disguises Sugar can take on? Sugar can and does go by many names. All of these should be avoided. Here are several examples of hidden sugars.

Sugar by Any Other Name Is Still Sugar

Barley malt	Beet sugar	Brown sugar
Buttered syrup	Cane juice crystals	Cane sugar
Caramel	Corn syrup	Corn syrup solids
Confectioner's sugar	Carob syrup	Castor sugar
Date sugar	Demerara sugar	Dextran
Dextrose	Diastatic malt	Diatase
Ethyl maltol	Fructose	Fruit juice
Fruit juice concentrate	Galactose	Glucose
Glucose solids	Golden sugar	Golden syrup
Grape sugar	High-fructose corn syrup	Honey
Icing sugar	Invert sugar	Lactose
Maltodextrin	Maltose	Malt syrup
Maple syrup	Molasses	Muscovado sugar
Panocha	Raw sugar	Refiner's syrup
Rice syrup	Sorbitol	Sorghum syrup
Sucrose	Sugar	Treacle
Turbinado sugar	Yellow sugar	

Fat – The Good, Bad and Ugly

So I bet you are wondering why you should up your fat consumption when you are trying to lose fat. Actually there are a number of factors at work here that will help you lose weight and maintain good health without restricting fat consumption.

First and foremost, your body needs fats to function properly. Fats are a central component of your nervous system. They are also key to helping your body absorb Vitamins A, D and E.

In order to get the adequate amount of calories and nutrients for your body to function properly, since you are eating significantly fewer carbohydrates you will by default need to increase your intake of fats.

There is no *real* reason for you to consume more fat on a Ketogenic Diet, since ketosis can easily be achieved by low carbs and high proteins. However, for your body to not to lose metabolism from a lack of calories (and thereby requiring you to reduce calories even more), fat in your diet is necessary to outweigh the loss of calories from carbs and to not get all of your calories from proteins.

Additionally, since many protein food groups contain fats, you would be severely restricting the number of food choices you have available to you. Dietary fats also help the taste of many proteins and help you feel full and satisfied.

Of course, like the other macronutrients (carbohydrates and proteins) there are the good, bad and ugly fats. Similar to carbs; enjoy the good, avoid the ugly and eat the bad sparingly (less than 10%).

Following is just a sampling of the ***Good, Bad and Ugly Fats*** you will find as you are planning your diet.

Finding the Good in Fat

Good Fats	Bad Fats	Ugly Fats
peanut butter	fat-dense meats	deep-fried foods
almond & cashew butter	bacon OK	processed meats
olives, black or green	poultry	foods fried in fats; donuts, french fries,
nuts – almonds, pecans, pistachios, cashews, brazil nuts, filberts, macadamia, walnuts, pine nuts	whole and 2 percent milk	most processed foods – check the label for fat content; if 'low fat' check for high sugar content
avocado	cheese	shortening
oils – olive, sesame, peanut, ~~canola~~, corn, cottonseed, flaxseed, grape seed, safflower, ~~soybean~~, sunflower	butter	margarine
fish: salmon, mackerel, herring, tuna	sour cream	any fats that turn solid
wild-caught fish	whipped cream	processed chips, crackers, cakes & cookies
grass-fed beef	whole cream	
free-range chicken	coconut oil OK	
seeds – pumpkin, sunflower, sesame, flaxseed	~~palm oil~~	

CHAPTER 4- WHAT YOU CAN EXPECT FROM THIS DIET

Superb Results Are Achievable

The Ketogenic Diet can help you lose unwanted fat and significantly reduce body weight, cholesterol and triglycerides. Many individuals have experienced better moods and heightened clarity in thinking. As with any controlled weight loss you can and should feel more energy.

One of the ideal benefits of this diet is that so many individuals find that they do not feel hungry after eating these types of foods. Not only is this very satisfying but it also makes it much easier to continue on the diet plan.

If you do this diet consistently, you can be sure that you will see great results. In fact, you are most likely to succeed with this diet if you take a holistic attitude and seek long term success with this diet program. By having a holistic attitude towards this diet program it means that you should have the right mindset, excellent nutrition, and the right foods – to make this program work for you.

While some see this dietary program as restrictive, it is one that is more of a very relaxed nature. You should quickly find out that the food choices are very delicious and satisfying. While you will be cutting carbs and as a result calories, you will feel full from the foods you are eating.

Even More Benefits

You will have less excess water weight because these foods will help your body pass this out on a regular basis. Low aldosterone, low insulin, drop in the level of muscle glycogen, will lead to a lot of excretion of both intra and extracellular fluids. BUT - this is really good news as this means hard and defined muscularity and results that are very quick and very clearly visible.

You get a bonus too as ketones give only 7 calories per gram. Better still is the fact that they cannot be converted back into the form of fatty acids. So any excess of ketones in the body are excreted by the body in the form of urine.

Another great plus is that the human brain just loves ketones and so in the state of Ketosis, you would tend to feel more positive, alert and clear headed.

Plus, as there will never ever be a shortage of supply of fats to ketones, you are going to have high energy levels at all times.

You will even feel like sleeping less as a result of this diet. But though you will sleep less, you will wake up feeling very refreshed – and all due to you being in a state of Ketosis.

If you combine this diet plan with good and regular exercise it is possible to see even better results. Many choose do engage in weight lifting to build muscle strength and tone the body.

The bottom line is that there are so many benefits that you can get from a Ketogenic Diet. Thus, if you are dreaming of having the best physique or low body fat figure, then this is just the type of diet that you should be doing.

Negative Perceptions About This Diet

There are some people who have negative things to say about this diet, in spite of the fact that this diet is a proven success for many people. When you begin this diet, it might be possible for you to experience slight discomforts like: fatigue, hunger, irritability or headaches. But the good news is that these will only last for 2 to 7 days.

Beginning anything new in life is not always easy and the same is the case with for the Ketogenic Diet.

CHAPTER 5- NOT JUST ANOTHER DIET

One thing you can be sure of is that the Ketogenic Diet is *not just another diet*. You can also be sure of this fact – all diets require a certain amount of change, discipline and patience – and the same is true with this type of diet. In addition to the discipline and patience, you would also need to watch your calorie intake and monitor the protein, fat and carbohydrates of the foods you eat.

Keep in mind that though we are all equal, no two bodies are the same and so what works for someone else, is not necessarily going to work for you. Simply put, if you want to make this diet work for you, you have to keep the specific needs of your body in mind.

How Do You Lose All The Extra Fat?

As you well know, there are some vehicles that run on gasoline and some that run on diesel. But what if you had a vehicle that would let you choose whether you want to run it on diesel or whether you want to run it on gasoline?

This would be real cool wouldn't it? In this way, if the price of gasoline rises, you can run the vehicle on diesel. And if the price of diesel rises, you can run the vehicle on gasoline. Now how awesome would that be!

Do you know that the human body is very akin to that of any vehicle, in the sense that just like a vehicle, the human body too needs fuel to run? Most of us get this fuel for our bodies from carbohydrates.

But the exciting part is that instead of using carbs to generate fuel for your body, you can get your body to make use of all the extra and unnecessary fat that you have stored in your body.

Use Fats and Proteins, Not Carbs to Get Energy and Nutrients

Your body is extremely efficient at finding and converting sources of fuel to energy in your body. If there are easily convertible sources such as carbs, it will use that and store the excess as fat for later. But if there are no carbs available it will convert fats and proteins to energy – the benefit here is that these sources require more energy and time to convert and the excess is not stored as fat.

That alternative fuel usage is just what the Ketogenic Diet is really all about. It is all about you telling your body to start making use of fats to produce energy for you. And in order for this to be accomplished you must start to consume more fats and proteins, while at the same time eliminating carbs from your diet – in fact, the less carbs you eat, the better it is going to be for you.

Lose That Extra Fat

The reason for you going on this Ketogenic Diet is very simple – because you want to get rid of that extra fat in your body. True, to be successful with this diet plan, you will need to consume large amounts of proteins and fats.

But this is the great part about this diet – your body will burn all this extra fat that you consume and in this way you will be able to get rid of all that fat that you are desperate to lose - and look and feel great.

Cycle in More Carbs on Specific Days

This simply means that when you are on this diet you can choose to have a number of days, typically 2 to 5 days per week where you can eat more carbs. So if you are a carb lover and find that you still crave carbs, you are definitely going to love this diet.

You can add in more carbs on these days, but need to make sure that your body does not go out of ketosis. If you choose to add in carb days, start with 2 days to see if your body still is able to return to at fat burning phase after the 2 days.

Later, you can up the number of carb days if your body is still able to stay in the Ketogenic state. Just be sure that you only do this on specified days and do not add more carbs during the other days.

Planning Your Meals

In fact, the truth is that the hardest part about this diet is planning out all your meals. You need to adhere to the following guidelines when you are on this diet plan:

- 60% – 70% Fats
- 30% Proteins
- 0 – 10% Carbohydrates

You can vary these amounts within the ranges in order to be able to eat foods you enjoy. While this is what you should aim at ideally, you will find that this is easier than you think! In Chapter 8 we will show you the wide variety of foods you can eat with your diet and in unlimited amounts.

You will be able to *eat as much as you would like* of these recommended foods because they aid in your fat burning. The trick here is that 'as much as you like' in reality isn't an excessive amount because these foods satisfy you and fill you up much sooner than high carb foods.

The above percentages are based on what is an acceptable percentage of the required calorie intake that your body needs. This also takes into account the percentage of body fat and the calculations of lean body mass that you are aiming to achieve.

Aside from the actual diet itself, the difficult part is sticking to what you can and cannot eat when you are on this diet. Additionally you will have to keep count of all the calories and the percentage of fat, protein and carbs that you are having daily.

You may find it easier to have a nutrient and calorie counter so you know what you have to eat and what you must not per meal – this will make the diet much easier for you to adhere to. You can of course follow our suggested guides later on in this book.

The point is that no matter what diet you plan to go on, it is going to take some counting of food intake and the same is the case with the Ketogenic Diet. But one thing you can be sure of with this diet, it is very different from the other diets and if you do it in the right way – it actually does work wonders for you.

CHAPTER 6- WILL YOU REALLY LOSE WEIGHT

This is a normal question for anyone to ask when they want to go on a diet - Am I going to lose weight if I go on this diet? But when you go on a Ketogenic Diet, have no doubt about the fact that not only are you going to lose weight – you will lose weight quickly.

Another big plus with this diet is that it gives you all the principles that you need for keeping in great shape and staying healthy and fit for a long period of time. Better still, when you are on this diet, you know for sure that you are on a sensible plan for weight loss.

How You Can Lose Weight With Eating More Fat

This diet is low in carbs, moderate in proteins and high in fats and it has been designed in such a way that it will provide you with all the calories and proteins that you need to have in order for you to have a healthy weight and nourish your body.

The main aim of this diet is to make the body burn excess fats and use these fats to fuel the energy that is required by the body – instead of making the body use carbohydrates for fuel. This is just great as in this way all the fats in the body are being burnt and this in turn helps greatly in promoting substantial weight loss.

There are many people who just recoil from the very thought that this is a diet that has high fat content. This is because most people normally associate fats with something that is unhealthy and bad for the body.

But this kind of thought process is somewhat misleading. This is because there is something that is known as "healthy fats" and these are very vital to many of your body functions.

Please make note of the fats I have shown you in *Good, Bad and Ugly Fat Chart* and choose your fats accordingly. Remember that good fats are an essential part of any healthy diet.

Will You Lose Weight?

Yes of course, when you are on this diet you are definitely going to lose weight – a lot of it in fact. And more, you can adopt the principles of having a low carb diet to ensure that you maintain a fitter and healthier lifestyle.

Rapid Weight Loss

Ketogenic Diets have created a strong following not just regular people but also with bodybuilders and famous athletes. Why? Because this diet can work for you! The Ketogenic Diet offers the opportunity to achieve fat loss very quickly while still maintaining muscle and toning your body.

When do this diet correctly, you will also be able to have greater muscle retention as compared to high protein (gluconeogenic) diets or even carbohydrate diets. You can also be very sure that not only will you actually see your fat loss, but you will also get high and very stable energy levels.

Get Started Right For Success

Start with a positive mental attitude. At first this diet can seem very restrictive and difficult. This can happen if you are not willing to change your eating habits periodically or try new foods and different food combinations.

However, we will soon show you the amazing variety of nutritious foods that will work well for you on this diet. There are also many food groups and recipes that you will soon see are very delicious and will also cause you to crave less sugar and carbohydrates.

Achieving Weight Loss With Any Weight Loss Program

Almost any weight loss program that you would enroll in, would tend to focus on either one of the following:

1. The intake of the 3 most vital macronutrients - namely carbohydrates, fats or proteins
2. Reduction of calories

This would be in order to enable you to achieve optimum weight loss. But when you go on the Ketogenic Diet, you can achieve weight loss quickly. This is because as soon as you go on this diet, your body will start going through various changes.

CHAPTER 7- HOW TO LOSE ALL THAT WEIGHT

Well of course you want to lose weight and you wanted to lose it yesterday right? How about if we just get started today instead. What I am going to talk about next should get you very excited because you can begin to drop that weight quickly.

> ❝ *If I had wanted to Diet,*
> *I wouldn't have*
> *eaten in the first place...*
>
> *Source Unknown*

What Weight You Should Expect To Lose

The initial weight loss, like many diets, will mostly be from excess water weight. For a 200 pound person, you may see as much weight loss as *6 pounds within the first 2 days*.

While this initial weight loss is mostly water, it helps you know that you are on the right track and your body is responding correctly to your new diet. This clearly will be also very motivating to you.

Then with you being on the diet for only 24 to 48 hours, your body will start to make use of ketones. The ketones enable your body to use the fat that is stored in your fat cells for energy. In this state you can achieve weight loss much more quickly.

Your body will continue to melt away these fats as you continue on your new diet plan. You should see anywhere *from ¼ of a pound to 2 pounds of weight loss per day*. These amounts will vary from person to person based upon what weight you started at, your insulin resistance, your food choices and other factors.

Let's Talk About Calories

We are very used to talking about calories and reducing calories for many of the diets we have tried and failed at or read about in almost any diet book and magazine. For many of us, this means a calorie restriction that becomes either impossible to stick to or most likely unrealistic to even begin trying.

The Ketogenic Diet will also talk about calories but in a way you are probably not used to even thinking about. This diet is about changing the percentage of macronutrients (fats, proteins and carbs) of your calories in order to lose fat.

You can start by going with your daily recommended calorie intake to maintain your body weight. This is typically between 1800 to 2400 calories for a 'normal' adult. The trouble with this is what is 'normal'. Frankly, a 600 calorie swing can make a big difference in weight. There are also differences for men and women and the amount of exercise or lack of exercise you do typically.

There are a number of ways you can apply your caloric intake with the Ketogenic Diet. First, you can start with your recommended 'maintenance' calories, but change the percentages from which nutrients those calories come from. Or, you could choose to reduce your caloric intake by a percentage or your daily recommended calories while still changing your macronutrient percentages.

I strongly recommend using a percentage of your recommended calories, instead of a fixed number of calories for a number of reasons. To begin with you should only reduce your total calories by a *maximum* of 20 percent.

For example, if your total maintenance calories are 2000 calories per day then the maximum amount of calories you should cut would be 400 (2000 x .20). This results in a new total calorie intake per day of 1600 calories (2000 – 400).

If you reduce your daily calorie intake below 20 % of your maintenance calories, you risk slowing your metabolic rate and thereby slowing your weight loss. Also, anything below this amount becomes extremely difficult to continue and increases the likelihood that you won't be able to follow your new diet plan.

I also recommend the percentage method because our bodies and lifestyles are all unique. You can always adjust these numbers once you know what works best for you to lose weight and stay on this diet.

How to Help Your Body Adjust

When you start this diet program, you need to first get your body into what is known as a "Ketogenic State". In order for you to get your body into this "state", you must go on a diet of low proteins, high fats and no carbs or hardly any carbs.

You could strive for a ratio of around 20% proteins and 80% fats to begin with for the first couple of days. This ratio should help you achieve ketosis more quickly. I personally do not follow this pattern, but some individuals can and do follow this. Again, just know you have choices and do what is right for you.

In my opinion a more ideal starting point is to still include a small percentage of carbohydrates and increase your intake of proteins and fats. These percentages allow for more variation in your food choices. If you have started your diet with the 20:80 percentages, then this will be stage two.

This is the suggested ratio of what you will be consuming:

- 10% carbs
- 30% proteins
- 70% fats

When you go on this diet it would mean that you would *reduce the amount of carbohydrates* that you consume. But at the same time, you would *be increasing the amount of proteins and fats* that you will consume. This is done so that you will be able to maintain the right muscle mass.

In general, when you go on this diet, you would have to abstain from consumption of all foods that are high in carbohydrates and these include foods like: bread, pasta, rice and potatoes. All of these foods are very high in carbohydrates.

Other foods you need to eliminate from your diet are the simple carbohydrates. These include sugars, fruit juices, honey and most all processed foods.

You just need to embrace the knowledge that fat will become your main source of energy and you will not need a large amount of carbs in your diet as an energy source.

How Many Carbs Is Low Carb?

To get your body in the fat burning mode you should consume less than 60 grams of net carbohydrates per day. Net carbs are the total carbohydrates listed minus the grams of carbohydrates from fiber.

When you look at ingredient labels if you do not see a net carb number, just subtract the fiber from the total carbs – this is the carb number you need to be concerned about.

As a general rule, in the beginning eat the least amount of carbohydrates your body can tolerate without losing energy or mental clarity. Fat and *not* carbs will become your main source of energy and any of these initial symptoms will disappear.

You can try starting with just 30 grams of net carbs per day and see how that works for you. You can then adjust your net carb intake as needed, but try not to consume more than 60 net carbs per day.

As you most likely have noticed by now, a little trial and error is needed with the percent of fats, proteins and carbs you will eat to arrive at what works best for your body. Each person is unique, so the nutrients required and resulting weight loss will vary from person to person.

The fact that you can make adjustments within the broader guidelines is actually ideal. In reality you will be doing what gets the best results for you and increases your ability to stick with this low carb diet.

CHAPTER 8- WHAT YOU CAN EAT TO MAKE THIS DIET WORK

Let us consider an example of how this diet works, note that these numbers are just being used for presentation purposes. You will need to determine your own maintenance calories and then follow these calculations.

A simple way to calculate maintenance calories is to take your current weight and multiply that by 15 – 17 calories. The result is the number of calories you can eat daily to maintain your current weight. Women should tend toward the lower end of the range and men the higher number.

If you want to lose weight, determine your goal weight and multiple that by 12 – 14 calories (20% less than maintenance calories) to get the daily calories required to lose weight. This has been a very good estimate for me of the daily calories I can eat to lose weight and still feel good.

There are also a number of online calorie counters available to use. You will find that these can give wild variances in the amount of recommended calories. We have some of these tools listed for you in our Resources Section at the end of this book. You can easily use these for you estimates. But do compare these calculations to the ones I show you here.

Just be sure you *don't decrease your calories too much* so that your metabolism slows down. You also don't want to set an unrealistic reduction in calories since this is so much harder to follow and sets you up for failure.

Jennifer Williams

Examples of How to Count Calories and Macronutrients

Let's say you weigh 170 pounds. To maintain this weight, without exercise, your daily recommended calories would be 170 lbs. x 15 kcal or 2550 calories daily.

You have two options here. You can stay with the current amount of maintenance calories, 2550 calories daily, and just adjust the percentages of where your nutrients come from according to the Ketogenic Diet recommendations.

Because of the rebalancing of your macronutrients, even with choosing the maintenance level you should experience some weight loss.

The other option is to reduce your caloric intake by a certain percentage (no more than 20 percent) in addition to changing the percentage of fats, proteins and carbs you eat according to the guidelines.

Now let's say your goal is to lose weight. To start with, let's choose to decrease your calories by the maximum of 20%. Your new daily recommended calorie intake would be 2040 calories (2550 kcal x .20 = 510 kcal; 2550 kcal – 510 kcal = 2040 kcal).

Thus, if we calculate our new maintenance weight we have 2040 kcal / 15 kcal = 136 lbs. This would be your new target weight from low carb dieting.

Whichever option you choose, you are sure to see results because you will have lowered your intake of carbohydrates. Your body will burn fat stores which will help you lose weight. You will also feel more full and satisfied from the higher proteins and fats and therefore 'naturally' reduce your calorie intake.

As I have mentioned before, you can adjust these caloric amounts and the percentages of macronutrients to what works best for you for maximum fat loss.

Follow your diet plan and day after day, the fat in your body will be reduced and you will begin to have a great looking body – one that will make you feel good too.

Your Food Choices Play A Big Role In This Diet

Since you have embarked on the Ketogenic Diet, you will have cut down on the consumption of carbs. Because you will maintain your protein intake at about 30% of your calories, the major part of your diet will now consist of fats – good fats.

As your body will not have carbs to use as a source of energy, it will now look at getting the energy from fat sources. This phenomenon is at the core of the Ketogenic Diet – your body can be retrained to burn greater amounts of fat by decreasing its use of glucose found in carbohydrates.

Take a look at the protein and fat sources that are available to you on this diet. Not only are the choices amazing and satisfying but, from the example list below, I hope you can see the vast number of options available to you to eat.

Isn't this a wonderful choice of foods that you can eat an unlimited amount of in your daily menu plan. As you look at these foods, can you see yourself over-eating any (many) of these foods? Of course not! This is why when I said previously that you will naturally find yourself reducing your daily calories it is because of the foods that you can eat on this diet.

All You Can Eat Foods

Beef	Steak	Hamburger
Prime Rib	Filet Mignon	Roast Beef
Chicken	Turkey	Duck
Fish; Tuna, Salmon, Trout, Halibut	Shellfish; Shrimp, Crab, Lobster, Oysters, Abalone	Lamb
Veal	Pork	Bacon
Ham	Bison	Eggs
Spinach	Lettuce	Mustard Greens
Vegetables (except potatoes)	Celery	Cucumbers
Avocado	~~Hummus~~	Olives
Nuts	Seeds	~~Condiments, unsweetened~~
~~Dairy~~	Butter	~~Cheese~~
Herbs	Oils; Olive, Sesame, ~~Peanut~~, ~~Canola~~, Flaxseed, ~~Safflower~~	Salt & Pepper

Of course, there are also foods that you can eat but you should enjoy them in more limited amounts. These foods are a good source of protein and good fiber. They also provide vitamins and minerals that our bodies need.

Limited Quantity Foods

Fruit (2 servings)	Berries -All types	Oranges
Lemons	Limes	Apples
Nectarines	Peaches	Melons
Bananas	Pineapples	Mangoes
Grapes (very limited)	~~Cottage cheese~~	~~Yogurt~~
~~Legumes~~	Beans	Peas
~~Mushrooms~~	Onions	~~Peppers~~
~~Sweet potatoes~~	~~Yams~~	

Last but not least...**Avoid All Sugars**. This includes sugar, breads, pasta, rice, potatoes, wheat, cornstarch, sauces or condiments with hidden sugars, and the vast list of ingredients that really are a sugar. Hint: if it ends in –ose it is a sugar.

Getting The Right Nutrients

As with any nutrition program or diet, you need to make sure you are getting the right nutrients to support your body's basic functions. The examples of food choices that we have shown you can give you these nutrients, just make sure that you eat a variety of these foods. Or, check out our Resources for great places to find individual nutrition content.

Keep in mind that the ratio of protein to fats intake should be around 1 to 2 with protein staying fairly constant at around 30 percent of your daily nutrients. This results in approximately 30% protein and 60% fats daily with the remainder 10% in carbohydrates. If you choose to reduce your carbs even further, increase your fats not your proteins.

It is a must for you to consume fats when you are on this diet. You have to consume fats as they will help you in fuelling your body and this in turn will help you in burning your body fat.

The good part about consuming fats is that it takes a long time to digest fats, so you will not feel hungry. As the digestion of fats is a slow process, it will be to your advantage as in this way you will feel "full" – instead of feeling hungry.

Certain Facts You Should Know About This Diet

At the start of this diet, you may feel drained of energy and slightly foggy for a few days while your body adjusts to metabolizing fats and proteins instead of carbohydrates. Just be aware that these feelings should be gone after the first few days.

If you are on the Ketogenic Diet for bodybuilding or body sculpting, you need to consume much more proteins than what you would normally do. This is because as you are limiting carbs you need to have proteins so that you will not lose any muscle tissue. Try to have around 5 to 6 meals per day or 3 meals with 2 snacks – with servings of protein included with all the meals that you are having.

As such, in the initial stages of this diet most proponents of this diet do not recommend you starting a new vigorous training program. Though a Ketogenic Diet is just great for bodybuilding or for weight loss, you have to make sure that you are consuming the right nutrients – if you do not, you will end up losing muscle mass.

More Proteins And More Fiber Too

Plus, as with any healthy diet you need to ensure that you are getting sufficient fiber. Since you want to lose that dirty fat that has built up within you, make it a point to get sufficient amounts of fiber to help clean your system.

You should find it easy to get fiber from your food selections. Here are some examples of good fiber sources.

Good Fiber Sources

Raspberries	Pear, with skin	Apple, with skin
Banana	Orange	Strawberries
Artichoke	Green peas	Broccoli
Turnip greens	Brussels sprouts	Sweet corn
Carrot, raw	Split peas	Lentils
Black beans	Lima beans	Baked beans
Almonds	Pecans	Pistachio nuts
Sunflower seed kernels		

So now that we have laid the basis of what you can and cannot eat and what core nutrients you need to be healthy, let's dive in to the mechanics of how you can plan your daily Ketogenic Diet.

CHAPTER 9- HOW TO PLAN AND START YOUR DIET

Okay, so now you know what how the fundamentals of how the Ketogenic Diet works. You also have a good idea of the percentage of fats, proteins and carbs you should eat daily. I have also shown you some examples of the variety of foods you can eat with your diet. Now, let's put this all together and have an actionable diet plan. Here is what you need to know to get started:

1. Start. Yes...Start. The problem with many diets is that we read about them and never actually *start* them. How many times have you waited for the 'right day' to start your diet, but not surprisingly that day never comes. Start today.
2. Have a plan. Know what meals you are going to eat and when. Have specific food items or recipes written down and ready to go. Make a list for the grocery store, farmers market or garden.
3. Get the food items that you will need for your meals. I find it works best to plan out about 3 days of meals. This is because most of the items you will eat are fresh meats, fish, vegetables and fruits.
4. Clear the refrigerator, cupboards, tables, desks, etc. of anything that does not fit into the items you planned in 2 and 3. Get rid of the things that do not fit into a low-carb lifestyle. Now, if you are like me I know that I won't waste food if at all possible. If so, either give them away or hide them – and I mean *really* hide them.
5. Measure, measure, measure. If you don't already have these items, get a food scale and measuring bowls, cups and spoons.

6. Get some storage containers. These are great if you want to make your meals in advance and store them for later. They are also great if you want to pack foods to take with you.

Remember, no matter what diet you decide to go on, it takes a great deal of dedication to stick with the diet. The same is the case with this diet plan. It is a bit tough for most people to abstain from eating carbohydrates all through the week. But bear in mind that you will be greatly rewarded for your dedication of starting, planning and sticking to this diet.

Menu Ideas for Your Main Meals

Here are just a few suggestions for the types of foods you could eat at each meal. This should give you an idea of the variety of menu items you can eat while still keeping within the diet guidelines.

Breakfast:

Eggs; scrambled, boiled or poached

Scrambled eggs with some parsley, tomatoes, spinach or scallions

Omelet with mushrooms, spinach and cheese

Bacon

Canadian bacon

Protein drink with fresh berries

Lunch:

Lettuce salad, with diced/sliced eggs, bacon and vegetables

Spinach salad with bacon and blue cheese crumbles

Salmon, tuna or chicken; alone or added to your salad

Cottage cheese with cucumbers or celery

Dinner:

Steak

Hamburger (no bun)

Chicken

Turkey

Fish

Vegetables, steamed or stir fried

Side Salad

Snacks:

Seeds

Nuts

Hardbolled egg

Cheese slices

A big reason for the success of this diet is because you have a variety of very delicious foods available to you. Thus, for as long as you are on this diet, you should never feel a sense of being deprived of eating good foods and neither should you feel hungry or unsatisfied.

Example Daily Menus

So now let's show you what this actually might look like with our chosen daily calorie intake and the recommended percentage of fats, proteins and carbs.

These are just a sampling of meals that I chose from my collection to give you a sense of what combinations you will be able to eat. Please keep in mind that these are just example and the calculations are approximate.

For our examples we are going to stick with our 2040 calorie per day target that we arrived at in Chapter 8 and make some adjustments in calories from there. I think you will be pleasantly surprised at the quality, variety and amount of delicious foods you can eat when you 'Kick The Carbs'.

2040 Calories per Day Example			
Breakfast:	**Quantity:**	**Total**	**Percent**
Omelet with goat cheese and bacon	2 (4 eggs)	2030 Calories	
Reduced fat milk	1 cup		
Lunch:		60g Carbs	11%
Cucumber and tomato toss	¾ cucumber, 1 ½ tomatoes	137g Fat	60%
Pecans	1 ounce	147g Protein	29%
Nonfat Greek Yogurt	6 ounces		
Dinner:			
Seared Strip Steak	5 ounces		
Asparagus with sliced almonds and parmesan cheese	½ pound asparagus		
	1 ½ ounces almonds		
	1 ½ ounces parmesan cheese		

To lower the daily calories to 1800, I have reduced the size of the Breakfast Omelet to 3 eggs and the size of Cucumber and Tomato salad for Lunch.

1800 Calories per Day Example			
Breakfast:	**Quantity:**	**Total**	**Percent**
Omelet with goat cheese and bacon	1.5 (3 eggs) *	1810 Calories	
Reduced fat milk	1 cup		
Lunch:		52g Carbs	11%
Cucumber and tomato toss	1/2 cucumber *, 1 tomato *	121g Fat	60%
Pecans	1 ounce	135g Protein	29%
Nonfat Greek Yogurt	6 ounces		
Dinner:			
Seared Strip Steak	5 ounces		
Asparagus with sliced almonds and	½ pound asparagus		
parmesan cheese	1 ½ ounces almonds		
	1 ½ ounces parmesan cheese		

Taking this one step further, we can reduce our daily calories to 1600 by again reducing the size of our Breakfast Omelet to 2 eggs and eliminating the Nonfat Greek Yogurt from Lunch.

1600 Calories per Day Example			
Breakfast:	**Quantity:**	**Total**	**Percent**
Omelet with goat cheese and bacon	1 (2 eggs) *	1590 Calories	
Reduced fat milk	1 cup		
Lunch:		44g Carbs	11%
Cucumber and tomato toss	1/2 cucumber, 1 tomato	112g Fat	62%
Pecans	1 ounce	107g Protein	27%
Nonfat Greek Yogurt	6 ounces		
Dinner:			
Seared Strip Steak	5 ounces		
Asparagus with sliced almonds and	½ pound asparagus		
parmesan cheese	1 ½ ounces almonds		
	1 ½ ounces parmesan cheese		

And finally, we can lower the daily Calories to 1400 by eliminating Pecans from our Lunch.

1400 Calories per Day Example			
Breakfast:	**Quantity:**	**Total**	**Percent**
Omelet with goat cheese and bacon	1 (2 eggs)	1390 Calories	
~~Reduced fat milk~~	1 cup		
Lunch:		40g Carbs	11%
Cucumber and tomato toss	1/2 cucumber, 1 tomato	91g Fat	59%
~~Pecans~~	~~1 ounce~~	105g Protein	30%
~~Nonfat Greek Yogurt~~	~~6 ounces~~		
Dinner:			
Seared Strip Steak	5 ounces		
Asparagus with sliced almonds and ~~parmesan cheese~~	½ pound asparagus		
	1 ½ ounces almonds		
	1 ½ ounces parmesan cheese		

As you can see from the examples, I have kept the menu items the same while adjusting either the quantities or eliminating items to lower the calories while still staying within the recommended percentages for fats, proteins and carbs. The quantities I have changed are highlighted with an * and items eliminated are crossed out.

CHAPTER 10- CYCLE IN SOME CARB UP DAYS

In the previous chapter we discussed the options available to you if you choose to go on a daily Ketogenic Diet. Another option you may choose – especially if you are a bodybuilder, athlete or like higher intensity activities – is to cycle in carbs on specific days.

The Cyclical Ketogenic Diet (CKD) suggests that you follow the Standard Diet for 5 days and then cycle in carbs on 2 days. If you engage in activities that could deplete your muscle stores faster, then this may be a good option for you. On the 2 days that you can load up on carbs, your muscles will have a chance to replenish themselves faster.

The CKD is also a good option for those individuals who are 'carb-addicts' and find the daily restrictions in carbs to be too hard to follow and stick to the diet. When you are following the CKD there is a special two day regimen where you can eat all the carbs that you love enjoying. Think of this as a 'reward' for your fat loss and following the carb restrictions all week long.

Monday to Friday, you will follow the above rules for this diet that you will be on. And then over the weekend, you will "carb-up". This "carb-up" process will start after you are through with your final workout on Friday.

During this "carb-up" stage that you will undergo over the weekends, you would be free to eat anything that you want, including foods like: pasta, pizza, breads and even ice-cream. The reality is that by eating such foods you are actually helping yourself by giving your body a boost and refueling your body for the week to come. But after the weekend is over, you are back to the "high fat, moderate protein, no carb diet".

The Right Time For You To Load Up On Carbs

The ideal time for you to start loading up on carbs is on Friday after 6 in the evening. And you should keep on consuming carbs till it is midnight on Sunday.

Perhaps you are thinking this – is there a limit to the amount of carbs that you should consume over the weekend? Well the answer to this one is really not at all easy.

Some people eat all that they want and they are able to get that correct balance of glycogen. But for others, there is a little bit of calculating that has to be done, so here goes the math…

For every lean kilogram of body mass that you have, the standard recommendation is that you need to take in around 10-12 grams of carbs. Thus, if you had 180 pounds of lean body mass – if you divide this by 2.2, you would get 82 grams of carbs. Not as hard as you would imagine it to be!

Alternative Number of Carb Days

Don't want to go low carb for 5 days? Then reduce your number of days for low carb and increase the carb up days. Just on those low carb days, stick to the diet plan wholeheartedly.

Bottom-line; this diet is about helping you to lose weight. If that means adjusting some things within the guidelines, please do so if that makes it easier to stick to your diet. Everyone's body is different and yours will tell you what is working and what isn't.

Modify It – Change It – Enjoy It

Make It Work For You

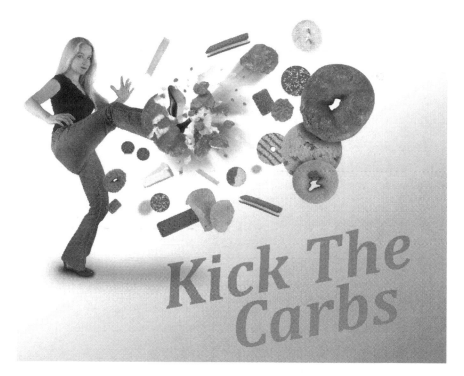

CHAPTER 11- ENDING THE KETOGENIC DIET

This is the big question for most people, even before they go on a diet – when will they be able to stop. Many people do not want to stay on this diet or any diet for the rest of their lives.

The main thing that you need to understand about the Ketogenic Diet is that mostly it is used by people to reach specific weight goal or muscle tone– be it for weight loss or for weight gain.

However, I have found that with the food choices I have and recipes that I am able to make, this low carb diet is very easy to continue for a long time. People find that the meals you can eat are delicious and leave you feeling full and satisfied.

To understand whether you can be on this diet for the rest of your life or not, all you have to do is ask yourself this simple question – just what would you say is a normal diet? Is it the kind of food that has simple carbs? Or is it junk food? Or is it some other kind of unhealthy food? The point here is that you should deliberate on the effectiveness of the foods that you consume. Are these foods going to help you in achieving your long term plans of fitness and health?

On the other hand, when you are on this diet, it guarantees that you will get all the right foods that your body needs to keep you healthy and in perfect shape. You can feel confident that when you are on this diet you are not going to have any issues with long term maintenance

Of course, if you choose to stay on a low carb diet for the rest of your life you can be sure that you will be having all the tools that you need to mold your body in the way that you desire whether you want to put on pounds or lose some – the choice is all yours.

CHAPTER 12- TIPS FOR SUCCESS

A Few Tips To Help You Succeed With The Ketogenic Diet

As you are planning your Ketogenic Diet, the following guidelines and tips are going to be helpful to you...

> *The best Diet is
> the one you will
> actually follow...*

Don't reduce your calories too much from maintenance levels at the beginning. Your body needs sufficient calories to function properly. You also don't want to make your diet plan unrealistic.

Contrary to what you may have heard for a long time, it is necessary that you consume fats. Just remember to eat good fats. Never forget the fact that your body needs fuel in order to be able to function. Your body will require these fats as a fuel source.

Yes you will also be eating proteins, but these do not make for as great of an energy source. So, your body will start making use of the fats that are stored in your body, as a fuel source.

As such, in order to be able to bring about the state of ketosis, an alternate source of fuel is needed for the body. Consume fats that are healthy and unsaturated such as seeds, nuts, olives, avocados, to name a few. Check our earlier diagram for suggestions.

You need to know your carb limitations: All of our bodies have different needs. Some individuals who are on this diet will have to keep to a very strict, low carb intake and this means less than 20 grams of carbs in a day. But for other people on this diet, they will be able to very comfortably stay in ketosis by consuming anywhere between 50 to 100 grams of carbs daily.

Now the tough part here lies in knowing how much carbs you would require and the truth is that you would only be able to know of the same by trial and error.

Drink water: When you are on the Ketogenic Diet, it is more difficult for your body to retain water. Thus it is very vital that you ensure that you stay properly hydrated. Keep a bottle of water or two, close at hand so that you can keep drinking water all the time.

According to experts, it is recommended that men must take in at least 3 liters of beverages on a daily basis, to ensure that they are well hydrated when on this diet. For women, 2.2 liters daily is recommended.

Get smart about drinking alcohol. If you like to have an occasional drink or two, you can indulge yourself while you are on this diet. You should choose from unsweetened liquors like: tequila, cognac, vodka, whiskey, scotch, brandy, gin, rum and possibly a low-carb beer. Keep in mind that calories do matter when you are on this diet so make sure that you stay within calorie limits if you plan to have an alcoholic drink.

Experiment: Choose a variety of foods and plan to adjust your calories and fat, protein, and carb percentages that work for you and help you lose the optimum weight.

Plan ahead: Nothing can derail a diet faster than not knowing what to eat for your next meal or snack, or not having the right ingredients on hand to make something that fits well within your diet and your taste buds.

Find some great recipes and choose from the foods you enjoy. This will help you in sticking with your diet. There is such a variety of tasty and nutritious foods you can eat on this diet, you really can't go wrong.

Count, calculate, adjust and count again. I will apologize in advance for scaring off all of the math-o-phobes, but this is very important to ensure you are doing this diet correctly. If you want to see results, you will need to know what calories and the percentage of each macronutrient you are eating. After a while, you will know what to eat more easily and you won't have to count as much.

Patience is really the key: While you can expect to see very fast weight loss on the Ketogenic Diet, the process of losing weight is one that is very slow and time-consuming. Your body will be making adjustments and you will be making adjustments to your eating habits too.

So, do not expect miracles to take place overnight. Have patience and stick to the diet and you will see the results in due course - if you do the Ketogenic Diet in the way it is meant to be done.

RECIPES

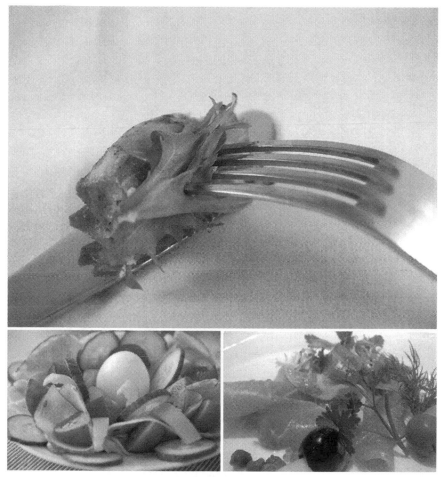

EGG AND BREAKFAST DISHES

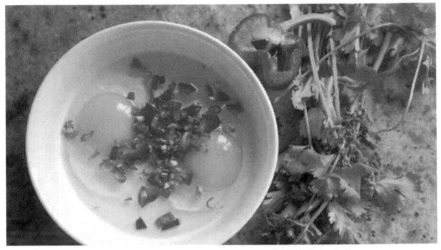

Breakfast is well touted as the most important meal of the day and rightfully so. Study after study has shown that children who eat breakfast perform better in school. Adults also perform better and are less likely to get over hungry and thus over eat.

What follows are some delicious and easy to make breakfast dishes that are low carb and give you the proteins and fats to start your day.

A good breakfast doesn't need to be complicated either. You can quickly make eggs – scrambled, boiled, or fried – add some bacon slices to the side and you are ready to go.

If you are crunched for time or just don't like to cook in the morning, grab a non-fat Greek Yogurt, a sliced avocado, a handful of nuts or a leftover slice of Quiche.

Just make sure you get a great start to your day!

Omelet with Goat Cheese and Bacon

Servings: 1

Prep Time: 5 Minutes

Cook Time: 10 Minutes

Per Serving: 252.4 Calories | 2.2g Carbs | 17.9g Fat | 20.3g Protein

INGREDIENTS:

2 extra large Egg

10 grams Goat cheese

1 slice Bacon, cut in small pieces

1 tbsp Onions, chopped

2 sprigs fresh Dill, chopped

1 pinch Salt and Pepper

DIRECTIONS:

Whisk the eggs with a pinch of salt and pepper to taste.

In a small frying pan, cook the bacon over moderately high heat until sizzling and partially cooked.

Pour the beaten eggs over the bacon; slightly turn the frying pan so the mixture covers the bottom of the pan; turn the heat to medium-low.

When the edges of the omelet start to harden slightly, sprinkle the cheese and onions evenly over the top of the omelet. When the eggs are almost stiff, sprinkle in the dill. Fold the omelet in half and cook until desired doneness.

Curry Cheddar Scrambled Eggs

Servings: 2

Prep Time: 5 Minutes

Cook Time: 10 Minutes

Per Serving: 235.4 Calories | 1.4g Carbs | 17.8g Fat | 17.7g Protein

INGREDIENTS:

4 extra-large Eggs

4 tbsp Cheddar cheese, shredded

1 tsp Butter

1/2 tsp Curry powder

Pinch of Salt and Pepper to taste

4 dash Pepper

DIRECTIONS:

Whisk the eggs. Add the curry powder, salt and pepper to the eggs; whisk together until well blended. Stir in the cheddar cheese. Melt the butter in a skillet over medium heat. Pour in the eggs and cook, stirring constantly until firm but still moist, 3 to 5 minutes.

Fluffy Omelet with Cheese and Spinach

Servings: 2

Prep Time: 5 Minutes

Cook Time: 10 Minutes

Per Serving: 544.5 Calories | 4g Carbs | 47g Fat | 28.5g Protein

INGREDIENTS:

6 extra large Egg

4 tbsp Butter

1 1/2 oz (6 tbsp) Cheddar cheese, shredded

2 tbsp chopped Chives

2 dash Salt

2 dash Pepper

12 leaf Spinach

DIRECTIONS:

Heat oven to broil. Separate egg yolks. Stir egg yolks together in a bowl. In a separate bowl, beat the eggs whites with a whisk or beater until soft peaks form. Fold the whites into the yolks.

Heat a 10 inch nonstick frying pan over medium heat and add butter. Once the butter sizzles, pour egg mixture evenly in the pan. Reduce heat to low and cook until set and golden brown (about 5 minutes).

Remove the pan from heat and sprinkle the top of the omelet with cheese, chives, salt, and pepper. Place omelet in frying pan under the broiler and cook until cheese melts, or 1-2 minutes. Remove frying pan from broiler, place spinach on top of cheese. Gently fold the omelet in half and serve.

Cheesy Asparagus and Ham Frittata

Servings: 2

Prep Time: 20 Minutes

Cook Time: 15 Minutes

Per Serving: 493 Calories | 5.5 Carbs | 34.7g Fat | 41.1g Protein

INGREDIENTS:

5 large eggs

8 medium asparagus stalks, trimmed and cut into 1/2 inch pieces

1/2 cup ham, finely chopped

4 tbsp freshly grated Parmesan

2 tbsp milk

1/4 tsp freshly grated lemon zest

1 tsp kosher salt

Freshly ground black pepper

1 tbsp extra-virgin olive oil

DIRECTIONS:

Preheat broiler with oven rack in top third of oven. Whisk the eggs; slowly add the 3 tbsp parmesan cheese, milk and lemon zest to egg mixture. Salt and pepper to taste.

Heat the olive oil in an 8-inch oven proof skillet over medium heat. Add the asparagus and ham; cook until the asparagus is crisp-tender

Reduce heat to low. Pour the egg mixture into the skillet; spread evenly over bottom of skillet. Cover and cook until the bottom sets up but does not brown - about 9 minutes.

Remove the cover. Sprinkle the remaining cheese over the top. Place the frittata under the broiler for about 1 minute, until slightly browned.

Let set for 5 minutes before removing from pan. Cut into slices.

MAIN DISHES – BEEF, PORK AND CHICKEN

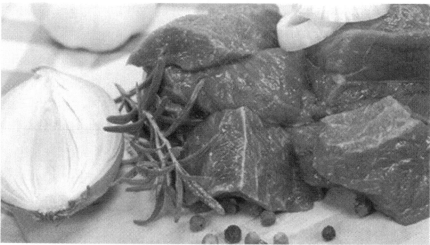

One of the great beauties of this diet is in the simplicity of meal preparation. This is especially true with the preparation of your main courses. A beautiful cut of meat, some healthy oils for cooking, add in some seasonings and dinner is served. What could be easier and more satisfying than that.

In the meat dishes here, you will find some added tidbits and ingredients that will make a favorite main course, like BBQ Ribs for example, work beautifully with a Low Carb, Ketogenic Diet without sacrificing flavor.

One of our favorite new finds is a wonderful ingredient that will enable you to bring a number of old recipes to a new 'low carb' life. Our new natural, high fiber ingredient has no protein, no fat, no sugar, no starch and no calories; it is also gluten free and wheat free. Sound interesting? Then dive in…

Beef Tenderloin with Garlic Butter

Servings: 2

Prep Time: 15 Minutes

Cook Time: 5 Minutes

Per Serving: 728.5 Calories | 1.1g Carbs | 62.5g Fat | 39.4g Protein

INGREDIENTS:

14 oz Beef tenderloin

4 tbsp Butter

1/3 clove Garlic, minced

1 large Scallion, chopped

1/2 tbsp Olive oil

1 dash Pepper

DIRECTIONS:

Place butter in a mixing bowl and using a fork, beat until soft. Add minced garlic and chopped scallions and mix. Spoon butter mixture onto plastic wrap and roll into a cylindrical-log shape. Refrigerate until firm (15 min).

Heat a frying pan over medium heat for 3-4 minutes until hot. Brush meat with olive oil and sprinkle with pepper. Place steaks in frying pan and cook without turning until juices rise to uncooked side, 1-2 minutes. Then turn over and cook to your desired doneness, 1 more minute for medium-rare or 2 minutes for medium to well-done.

Place steaks on serving plates, cut garlic butter into quarters and place one on each steak.

Just perfect served with a side salad.

Feta-Stuffed Hamburger

Servings: 4

Prep Time: 5 Minutes

Cook Time: 15 Minutes

Per Serving: 344 Calories | 1.8g Carbs | 25g Fat | 26.4g Protein

INGREDIENTS:

1 lb Ground beef

1/2 tsp Worcestershire sauce

1 tsp Parsley

1 dash Salt

1 dash Pepper

1 cup, crumbled Feta cheese

DIRECTIONS:

Preheat an outdoor grill for medium heat and lightly oil the grate.

Knead together the ground beef, Worcestershire sauce, parsley, salt, and pepper in a bowl. Form the mixture into 8 equal-sized balls; flatten to make thin patties.

Place 1/4 cup of the feta cheese onto four of the patties. Place the remaining four patties onto each of the patties prepared with the cheese; press the edges together to seal the cheese into the center.

Cook on the preheated grill until the burgers are cooked to your desired degree of doneness, 7 to 8 minutes per side for well done. An instant-read thermometer inserted into the center should read 160 degrees F (70 degrees C).

Kansas City Style BBQ Ribs

"If you love BBQ Ribs, you are going to be in for a real treat when you taste these ribs made with sauce from the famous Jack Stack Restaurant in Kansas City While ribs are made with the Low Carb version of their Famous Sauce, the flavor is so good you won't even know the difference. . .

Servings: 4

Prep Time: 10 Minutes

Cook Time: 1 Hour 30 Minutes

Per Serving: 520.5 Calories | 10.5 Carbs |19.3g Fat | 71.1g Protein

INGREDIENTS:

3 pounds Baby Back Pork Ribs

2 cups Jack Stack Low Carb BBQ Sauce (see Resource Section)

Dry Rub:

1 tbsp Kosher Salt

2 tsp Hungarian Paprika

2 tsp Garlic Powder

1 tbsp Parsley, dried

2 tsp freshly ground black, green and red peppercorns

DIRECTIONS:

Pre-heat oven to 350 degrees.

Cut the pork ribs into manageable portions; 4 – 5 Ribs per section is ideal.

Line 9x12 glass baking dish with tin foil. Add additional measure of foil to make a sealed pocket over the top of the ribs.

Mix together Dry Rub ingredients. Rub mix thoroughly into pork ribs. Lay ribs in bottom of foil-lined pan. Add 1/4 cup water to bottom of pan. Seal the tin foil tightly over the top of the ribs without touching the ribs; the foil should form a dome-shaped pocket over the ribs.

Roast ribs for1 hour. Remove ribs from oven and carefully open sealed tin foil over ribs. Baste ribs with the Jack Stack BBQ Sauce. Leave tinfoil unsealed and return ribs to oven for another 20 to 30 minutes; enough to flavor ribs but without turning sauce black. Serve immediately.

Beef and Bacon Rollups

Servings: 8

Prep Time: 20 Minutes

Cook Time: 50 Minutes

Per Serving: 245.6 Calories | 2.9 Carbs |11.7g Fat | 30.9g Protein

INGREDIENTS:

2 extra large Eggs

1/4 cup Ketchup

2 tbsp Worcestershire sauce

4 oz Cheddar cheese

1/4 cup Onions, chopped

2 tbsp Parmesan cheese

1 tsp Salt

1/4 tsp Pepper

2 lbs Ground beef

12 strips Bacon

DIRECTIONS:

Preheat oven to 375 degrees F. Line a baking sheet with heavy foil.

In a large bowl, combine all ingredients except the bacon. Mix well then shape in two 6-inch long log shapes.

On a large sheet of wax paper, lay 6 slices of the bacon side by side. Set one of the beef rolls crosswise at one end of the row of bacon strips; roll up, wrapping the meat with the bacon.

Place meat logs on baking sheet, seam side down. Bake for 45-50 minutes or until center reaches 160 degrees. Place under broiler 1 – 2 minutes to crisp and brown bacon, if needed.

Asian Chicken Lettuce Boats

Servings: 4

Prep Time: 5 Minutes

Cook Time: 15 Minutes

Per Serving: 232 Calories | 5.9 Carbs | 12g Fat | 25.7g Protein

INGREDIENTS:

2 tsp Canola Oil

8 oz Button Mushrooms, chopped

1 lb Lean Ground Chicken [319767]

1 clove Garlic, minced

1/2 tsp fresh Ginger, minced

1 cup Green Onions, sliced

1 8oz can Water Chestnuts, sliced

8 large Lettuce Leaves

1 tbsp Toasted Sesame Oil

1/2 tbsp Rice Wine Vinegar

3/4 tsp low-sodium Soy Sauce

1/2 tsp honey

Scallions, sliced for garnish

DIRECTIONS:

Heat canola oil in large nonstick skillet over medium heat. Add mushrooms and cook for 5 minutes or until tender; set mushrooms aside.

Add chicken, garlic and ginger to skillet and cook for 6-7 minutes or until chicken is brown, breaking the chicken into medium-small chunks. Tip: Use a potato masher to break up the ground meat.

Combine the chicken mixture with the cooked mushrooms; add green onions and water chestnuts; toss together. Combine sesame oil, rice wine vinegar, lower-sodium soy sauce, honey and crushed red pepper flakes in a small bowl; mix well.

Divide chicken mixture evenly between each lettuce leaves and top with sesame oil mixture. Garnish with scallions.

Slow Cooker Apricot Glazed Pork Roast

Servings: 8

Prep Time: 5 Minutes

Cook Time: 540 Minutes

Per Serving: 349.7 Calories | 8.8 Carbs |10.1g Fat | 53.5g Protein

INGREDIENTS:

11 oz Chicken broth

2 cups Low Carb Apricot Preserves – see Recipe Below

1 cup Onions, chopped

2 tbsp Dijon mustard

4 lbs Pork top loin roast

DIRECTIONS:

Mix broth, preserves, onion and mustard in 3 1/2-qt. slow cooker.

Add pork loin to cooker; cut in chunks to fit.

Cover and cook on low 8 to 9 hours or until done.

Low Carb Apricot Preserves

"This recipe can be used in a variety of dishes. Not only is this lower carb than store-bought preserves, but the nutritional value is exceptional; very high in Vitamins A and C, and Dietary Fiber, high in Potassium, and very low sodium

Yield: About 1 Cup

Serving Size: 1 Tbsp.

Prep Time: 5 Minutes

Cook Time: 0 Minutes

Per Serving: 13.4 Calories | 3.2 Carbs | 0.1g Fat | 0.4g Protein

INGREDIENTS:

2 small Nectarines, peeled

6 Apricots

1 – 1 1/2 tsp. Glucomannan Powder (Konjac powder)* (see Resource Section)

DIRECTIONS:

Remove seeds from apricots and nectarines; Cut into wedges.

Add apricots to blender. Coarsely blend; very slowly add (sprinkle) in Glucomannan Powder, starting with only 1 tsp. Add in Nectarines and continue blending and adding Glucomannan Powder until desired consistency.

(You can also substitute 1 large Peach for the Nectarines if desired.)

Note: the Glucomannan Powder is a high fiber thickening agent and can set up very quickly. The amount you add to your preserves will depend upon the juiciness of your fruits.

*Konjac Glucomannan Powder (see Resource Section) is a pure soluble fiber with no protein, no fat, no sugar, no starch and no calories; it is also gluten free and wheat free.

It has the highest level of viscous soluble fiber found in nature. With this higher viscosity of soluble fiber, you have better control over your blood sugar levels.

You can use the powder as a thickening agent in many sauces, gravies, and other recipes where you would have previously used cornstarch or flour. It has about 10 times the thickening power of cornstarch and as such, should be added to liquids and mixed well before adding to solids.

5 Minute Pepperoni Pizza

Servings: 4

Prep Time: 5 Minutes

Cook Time: 5 Minutes

Per Serving: 335.7 Calories | 6.8g Carbs | 25.3g Fat | 20.8g Protein

INGREDIENTS:

4 oz Pepperoni

8 oz Mozzarella cheese

2 cups Broccoli, chopped

DIRECTIONS:

Turn on oven broiler. Prepare a foil lined baking sheet. Lay 6 large slices of pepperoni, overlapping each other in a 3x2 formation, creating the "crust" of the pizza. Lay 1 oz of cheese on top of pepperoni; top with broccoli; add remaining cheese to top.

Place in oven, on rack nearest broiler. Broil for 5 minutes, until cheese is melted.

Chicken Stir Fry

Servings: 2

Prep Time: 15 Minutes

Cook Time: 15 Minutes

Per Serving: 410.5 Calories | 12.8g Carbs | 24.3g Fat | 34.7g Protein

INGREDIENTS:

1 Chicken breast, bone and skin removed

2 extra-large Eggs

1/2 Avocado, sliced

1/3 tbsp Coconut oil

4 ounces Asparagus

1 medium Red bell pepper

1 clove Garlic, minced

1/4 cup Almonds, sliced

DIRECTIONS:

In a small bowl, beat eggs and 3 tbsps. water together. Set aside.

Heat a large skillet over medium-high heat. When pan is hot, add coconut oil. Add asparagus, red pepper, and garlic; Sauté for 5 minutes, or until slightly tender.

Slice chicken into strips. Add chicken and eggs to vegetables. Cook, stirring constantly until vegetables are slightly tender, eggs are cooked, and chicken is cooked through. Season with sea salt (if desired), and top with almonds and avocado to serve.

MAIN DISHES – SEAFOOD

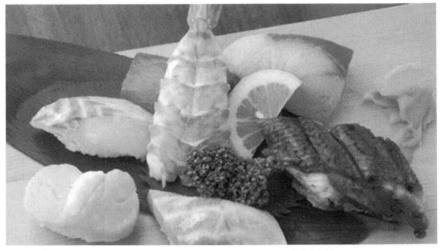

Fish and shellfish also offer an endless variety of delicious healthy dishes. Not unlike beef, pork and poultry, you can prepare an unlimited variety of mouth-watering appetizers, entrees and salads by just adding a few ingredients.

While the varieties of seafood are endless, just be sure you know what you are buying and from whom. In an ideal situation, you could just buy fresh seafood locally, but for many of us that is not possible all year round. Just be sure you are buying fresh or fresh frozen fish and seafood from a merchant you can trust so you are getting what you intended to eat.

Broiled Tilapia Parmesan

Servings: 2

Prep Time: 5 Minutes

Cook Time: 10 Minutes

Per Serving: 202 Calories | 1.5g Carbs | 10.7g Fat | 25.3g Protein

INGREDIENTS:

16 oz Tilapia

1/4 cup Parmesan cheese

2 tbsp Butter

1 tbsp Mayonnaise

1 tbsp Lemon juice

Seasoning mix:

1 tsp dried Basil

1/2 tsp Onion powder

1/2 tsp Celery salt

Pepper, pinch

DIRECTIONS:

Preheat your oven's broiler. Grease a broiling pan or line pan with aluminum foil.

In a small bowl, mix together the Parmesan cheese, butter, mayonnaise and lemon juice. Add seasoning mix from above (dried basil, pepper, onion powder and celery salt. Mix well and set aside.

Arrange fillets in a single layer on the prepared pan. Broil a few inches from the heat for 2 to 3 minutes. Flip the fillets over and broil for 2 to 3 more minutes.

Remove the fillets from the oven and cover them with the Parmesan cheese mixture on the top side. Broil for 2 more minutes or until the topping is browned and fish flakes easily with a fork; be careful not to overcook the Tilapia.

Salmon with Balsamic Vinaigrette

Servings: 2

Prep Time: 5 Minutes

Cook Time: 10 Minutes

Per Serving: 257.8 Calories | 1.1g Carbs | 17.4g Fat | 22.7g Protein

INGREDIENTS:

8 oz fresh Salmon fillet

1 dash Kosher Salt

2 tbsp Balsamic Vinegar

2 tbsp Olive oil

1 tbsp Lemon juice

1 clove Garlic, minced

Herbes de Provence, sprinkle to taste

{You can buy Herbes de Provence or use the Recipe that follows}

DIRECTIONS:

Combine kosher salt, balsamic vinegar, olive oil, lemon juice and fresh garlic in a small bowl. Coat salmon fillet on both sides with mixture. Place salmon skin side down in broiler pan. Sprinkle lightly with Herbes de Provence.

Broil salmon in oven 4" from broiler for 4-6 minutes or until the salmon flakes.

Maryland Crab Cakes

Servings: 4

Prep Time: 5 Minutes

Cook Time: 10 Minutes

Per Serving: 416 Calories | 4.6 Carbs | 23.7g Fat | 42.9g Protein

INGREDIENTS:

1 pound Crab Meat

4 oz bag of Pork Rinds, (snack-type) no added flavor, crumbled

1/4 cup Milk

1 Egg

3 tablespoons Mayonnaise

1 tablespoon Worcestershire sauce

1 teaspoon Mustard

2 Green Onions, sliced

1/4 teaspoon Salt

1/8 teaspoon Pepper

1 tablespoon Olive oil

1 tablespoon Butter

Optional: Glucomannan Powder (Konjac powder) for binding (see Resource Section)

DIRECTIONS:

Mix the crab, pork rinds, milk, egg, mayonnaise, Worcestershire sauce, mustard, green onions, salt and pepper in a bowl. You can add a sprinkling of Glucomannan Powder for binding, if needed.

Grab a handful of the mixture and form a rounded patty.

Heat the oil and melt the butter in a pan.

Jennifer Williams

Fry the patty in the oil and butter until golden brown on both sides, about 2-4 minutes per side.

Zesty Garlic Shrimp

Servings: 6

Prep Time: 10 Minutes

Cook Time: 10 Minutes

Per Serving: 245.6 Calories | 2.9 Carbs |11.7g Fat | 30.9g Protein

INGREDIENTS:

1 tsp Paprika

1/4 tsp Pepper

4 tbsp Basil, chopped

1/2 tsp Salt

1 clove Garlic, minced

1/4 cup Lemon juice

1/4 cup Olive oil

1 tsp Cayenne pepper

32 oz Shrimp

DIRECTIONS:

Heat the oil in a large skillet over high heat; cook and stir the garlic in the oil until translucent. Sprinkle the red pepper flakes and paprika into the oil.

Add the shrimp and toss to coat.

Pour the lemon juice over the shrimp; allow to cook until the shrimp are bright pink on the outside and the meat is no longer transparent in the center, 1 to 2 minutes more.

Reduce heat to medium-low; add the basil and toss lightly.

Season with salt and pepper.

Herbes de Provence

Yield: 1 Cup

Prep Time: 5 Minutes

INGREDIENTS:

2 tbsp dried Savory

2 tbsp dried Rosemary

2 tbsp dried Thyme

2 tbsp dried Oregano

2 tbsp dried Basil

2 tbsp dried Marjoram

2 tbsp dried Fennel seed

DIRECTIONS:

In a small mixing bowl, combine all the ingredients together. Store in an air-tight container

SALADS AND SIDE DISHES

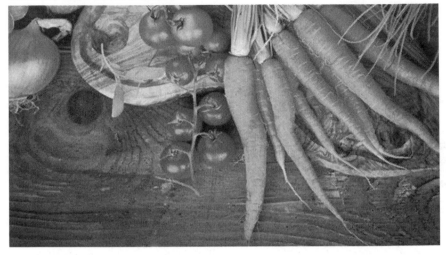

With salads, the variety and nutritional values are again easy and endless. Mixing up a salad with a multitude of 'diet-approved' vegetables and fruits is so easy. For vegetable side dishes, you can eat your favorite veggies raw or steamed, and simply add seasonings to taste.

In preparing salads, just be sure you use dressings or toppings that are low carb – the bottled salad dressings are a nightmare to navigate through their ingredients since they can contain a lot of sugar or an abundance of ingredients you can't even pronounce. Hint: if you can't pronounce it, you probably don't want to eat it!

If you can use fresh local produce or homegrown varieties all the better. You will find their taste is amazing and incredibly satisfying

Artichokes with Garlic Butter

Servings: 2

Prep Time: 5 Minutes

Cook Time: 20 Minutes

Per Serving: 182.6 Calories | 18.1g Carbs | 11.8g Fat | 5.6g Protein

INGREDIENTS:

2 large Artichokes

2 tbsp Butter

2 cloves Garlic, sliced

1 pinch Salt

1 pinch Pepper

DIRECTIONS:

Cover bottom of large stock pot with water. Bring water to a full boil over high heat. While water is heating, trim and discard the stems and tough outer leaves of artichokes. Tuck slivers of butter and slices of garlic into artichoke leaves.

When water is boiling, place steamer insert in pot and set artichokes in steamer, stem-side down. Cover pot with lid and allow artichokes to steam for approximately 20 minutes, until tender. Salt and pepper to taste.

Cucumber and Tomato Toss

Servings: 4

Prep Time: 15 Minutes

Cook Time: 0 Minutes

Per Serving: 91.6 Calories | 6.5 Carbs |7g Fat | 1.3g Protein

INGREDIENTS:

1 large Cucumber, cut into large cubes

2 large Tomatoes, cut into wedges

2 tbsp Balsamic vinegar

2 tbsp Olive oil

Salt

Pepper, freshly ground

Optional: minced garlic, fresh parsley

DIRECTIONS:

Place cucumbers and tomatoes in a bowl. Pour in olive oil and balsamic vinegar. Season with salt and pepper. Toss gently to coat. Refrigerate until ready to serve.

Roasted Cauliflower

Servings: 6

Prep Time: 10 Minutes

Cook Time: 25 Minutes

Per Serving: 145 Calories | 5.3 Carbs |10.2g Fat | 7.5g Protein

INGREDIENTS:

2 tablespoons minced garlic

3 tablespoons olive oil

1 large head cauliflower, separated into florets

1/3 cup grated Parmesan cheese

Salt

Pepper

1 tablespoon chopped fresh parsley

DIRECTIONS:

Preheat oven to 450 F. Grease a large casserole dish.

Place the olive oil and garlic in a large resealable bag. Add cauliflower, and shake to mix. Pour into the prepared casserole dish, and season with salt and pepper to taste.

Bake for 25 minutes, stirring halfway through. Top with Parmesan cheese and parsley. Broil for 3 to 5 minutes, until golden brown.

Asparagus with Sliced Almonds and Parmesan

Servings: 4

Prep Time: 2 Minutes

Cook Time: 10 Minutes

Per Serving: 154.2 Calories | 6.4 Carbs | 12.1g Fat | 7.4g Protein

INGREDIENTS:

2 tbsp Butter

1 lb Asparagus

1/3 cup Almonds, sliced

1/3 cup Parmesan cheese, freshly grated

DIRECTIONS:

Melt butter in a large skillet over medium-high heat. Add the asparagus, and cook about 3 minutes. Stir in almonds and parmesan, and cook until the cheese is slightly browned, about 3 to 5 minutes.

Chicken and Avocado Salad

Servings: 2

Prep Time: 5 Minutes

Cook Time: 20 Minutes

Per Serving: 403.6 Calories | 12g Carbs | 25g Fat | 34.6g Protein

INGREDIENTS:

9 oz boneless, skinless Chicken Breasts, cooked

1 Avocado

6 sprigs fresh Cilantro, chopped

1/2 Lime, squeezed for juice

8 large Lettuce leaves

Salt

DIRECTIONS:

Combine the chicken, avocado, cilantro, squeezed lime juice, and salt to taste. Let marinate for 10 minutes. Arrange the bib leaves, and serve the chicken salad on top.

Blue Buffalo Chicken Salad

Servings: 4

Prep Time: 20 Minutes

Cook Time: 15 Minutes

Per Serving: 449 Calories | 5.5 Carbs |28.4g Fat | 38.5g Protein

INGREDIENTS:

2 tbsp unsalted Butter, melted

1/2 cup Hot Sauce

1 1/4 pounds skinless, boneless Chicken Breasts

1 tbsp Extra-Virgin Olive Oil

1 cup Crumbled Blue Cheese

1/2 cup Sour Cream

4 stalks Celery, thinly sliced, plus 1/4 cup chopped celery leaves

1/4 small Red Onion, thinly sliced

1 Carrot, thinly sliced

1 head Iceberg Lettuce, cut into 4 wedges

DIRECTIONS:

Heat grill to high. Mix the melted butter and hot sauce. Brush chicken with olive oil. Grill chicken breasts basting frequently with butter and hot sauce mixture. Turn frequently to fully baste chicken and cook thoroughly. Remove from grill and let rest 5 minutes. Cut into bite size pieces. Toss with remaining hot sauce.

Puree 3/4 cup blue cheese and the sour cream in a blender until smooth. Add half of the blue cheese mixture to the chicken; add the sliced celery, celery leaves, red onion and carrot; toss.

Serve 1 lettuce wedge with 1/4 of chicken mixture. Drizzle remaining blue cheese dressing over top and sprinkle with blue cheese crumbles.

Chicken Salad with Toasted Almonds

Servings: 4

Prep Time: 5 Minutes

Cook Time: 5 Minutes

Per Serving: 292 Calories | 5.8g Carbs | 19.1g Fat | 24.9g Protein

INGREDIENTS:

2 cups cooked Chicken breast, cubed

8 tbsp Mayonnaise

1/4 tsp Pepper

1/2 cup, slivered Almonds, toasted

½ cup Celery, chopped

1 tbsp Lemon juice

DIRECTIONS:

In a large bowl, add almonds and celery to cubed chicken. Mix together mayonnaise, lemon juice, and pepper. Toss with chicken, almonds, and celery.

RESOURCES

Recommended Specialty Ingredients:

Jack Stack Low Carb BBQ Sauce – Buy here: http://amzn.to/118eZeR

Glucomannan Powder – Buy here: http://amzn.to/11YHvdZ

Calorie Counters:

The Mayo Clinic Calorie Counter – Calculate your daily calories needed to maintain your current weight.

http://www.mayoclinic.com/health/calorie-calculator/NU00598

Keto Calculator – Calculate your daily calories and intake of fats and proteins based upon the Standard Ketogenic Diet.

http://keto-calculator.ankerl.com/

Recipe Analyzers:

Calorie Count from About.com – Analyze your own recipes to determine calories, fats, proteins and carbs and standard nutritional content.

http://caloriecount.about.com/cc/recipe_analysis.php

Fruits and Veggies More Matters – Excellent nutrition database of thousands of fruits and vegetables. Find the full nutrition content of individual veggies and fruits. Learn how to select the best produce and properly store it. You will also find eating and preparation suggestions for your favorites.

Jennifer Williams

http://www.fruitsandveggiesmorematters.org/vegetable-nutrition-database

http://www.fruitsandveggiesmorematters.org/fruit-nutrition-database

ABOUT THE AUTHOR

Jennifer Williams spent a few decades working in large Multinational Corporations evaluating and improving business operations around the World. She was able to explore many different cultures and lifestyles during these travels. During one of her last excursions, she realized she knew more about the countries she visited and worked in than the city in which she called home. It was time to take another turn.

She left the 'ideal' career to spend time with family and friends and pursue her many interests. Now, she has spent the last decade cultivating these passions, many relating to home, food and health. She writes about many of these topics and is a syndicated contributor with the eMJayMedia network.

Jennifer is an exhaustive researcher and has hands-on experience with the topics she covers. Her books are designed to help people find inspiration and answers to questions they have in everyday life.

Jennifer currently resides in Madison, WI with her daughter, two cats, one dog, and an occasional horse...or two.

Made in the USA
Middletown, DE
22 October 2016